Exercise Exposed

Harrison Langdon Ennis

The Foundational Basics of Effective Exercise

Critical Information You Need to Know

Health Through Fitness Corrected

About The Author: Harrison Langdon Ennis

HLE is considered to be a true renaissance man of the twenty first century by many of his friends and associates. He is a published author and song writer/musician, as well as owning various design patents for products he markets. Has an affinity for bona fide dance music, and is a votary of shag dance. Realizing that life is a science, not a roll of the dice led him to serious research on the science of life for over a quarter of a century. Lifelong involvement in physical culture; to include martial arts, yoga, and traditional exercise, along with various obscure modalities. Former licensed private investigator, bodyguard and club bouncer, and training partner for a PKA World Champion.

Fitness / wellness researcher and coach, esoteric educator, and self- help life science counselor. A voracious tracker of cutting edge health products and practices. Past general manager for one of the largest health and fitness club facilities in a major metropolitan area.

His milestone expositions, **Life is a Science, Not a Roll of the Dice, Infinity of Intrigue, Yoga Compact** and other insightful books and essays attempt to synthesize and bring about greater understanding of the spiritual, mental, emotional, and physical aspects of life, how they operate in relation to each other, and offers information on how we, as individuals, can keep these aspects operating in harmony for the well-being of our total entity, and our future existence.

Proffers his **Yoga Life Science Regimen**™ and **Yoga by Ennis**™ as a personal trainer for individuals and groups, and gives seminar sessions by request and special arrangement. A firm advocate of meditation, proper nutrition, and physical exercise. Assesses these aspects as the primary keys for bringing forth our greatest potential, and for defining our ultimate purpose in life. He brings the wisdom of the ages to our modern dilemmas by offering techniques designed to negotiate a complete self-renewal process.

View other Cutting Edge Material, Services, and Products at:
www.hleproductions.com / www.selfhelplifestyle.com

"HLE is a man of several unique talents with a personality to match."

"In addition to helping people, that boy loves to shag dance."

"Loved, admired, and notorious in some circles."

"His mind works overtime."

By my own experience of testing, analyzing and experimenting with most exercise types that have come down the pike in the last 30 years, I recommend what is put forth in this material as being most effective. I would not use these protocols myself, if it were not so. They are techniques that you can sensibly and realistically implement into a Self Help Lifestyle.

In the final analysis of the modes presented, you will find no gimmickry. Directions will be simple to follow, and will require a small amount of time. It does not promote hours of cardio per week, and describes only the most result driven resistance exercise. It lays out the easiest, most feasible eating solution for fat loss, lean muscularity, and a leap in your health and fitness level relative to your exercise session. These scientific techniques will prove to be amazing in the way they can transform your life.

The material does not 'beat around the bush' relating pages of unnecessary scientific jargon. It presents the results of the science from top researchers around the world, and explains how to utilize the results. Interestingly, the lifestyle of our ancient forbearers jives right long with 21st century science. The truth about current general health and fitness regimens used extensively is brought to bear. It describes what does not work, what does work, and what to do.

Clamp down on this basic methodology, and quit spinning your wheels running around putting band-aids on all the variables that have to be corralled for the best results. Design free wheeling exercise that lends to creative expression of modality, and takes a small amount of time. Allow your body to burn fat, add muscle, ramp up strength and stamina, and upgrade your overall health, simultaneously, each day, with this basic, specific information!

Lack of a regular exercise program is believed to contribute to the death of over a quarter of a million people each year. Take exercise seriously. Not to do so is tantamount to slow suicide. This is one of the prerequisites to living a full life. Determine to master your fitness plan by knowledge, control, consistency, and pride. Make this area of your life a discipline and lifetime habit. It will stand you in good stead for the rest of your earthy sojourn.

Introduction

The Bible says, *"Know ye not that ye are the temple of God, and the spirit of God dwelleth in you."* This tells us that the great I Am's point of contact with the world is the physical body. Our physical vehicle has hidden significance that reaches far beyond its observable physical functions. It is an outpost of a bigger picture in which our higher and subtler aspects strive to advance. To hinder the health and duration of the physical body in this particular sojourn on earth, not only makes for a less pleasant existence, but also stunts the growth of our consciousness. If we hone in on spiritual matters exclusively, we are neglecting our physical roots, which can bring harmful repercussions. We should recognize that there is a circuitous rate of vitality between spirit and physicality.

Just as we have to keep our automobile in proper condition by preventative maintenance, to serve us, and reach various destinations, we have to do the same thing with our physical body. The well-functioning and capable physical body enables us to operate properly and efficiently in our daily affairs, which may include a variety of things such as working, learning, recreation, thinking, socializing, sex, and so on, as well as enabling our consciousness to expand.

So, the basic thing that we want exercise to do for us is to improve our functional abilities. Exercise of almost any kind, properly done, has a positive effect on the physical body and our inner, subtle aspects. It is a wonderful tool to center and ground you. It has a rational and calming effect on your feelings and emotions. However, its major effect is to keep you strong, flexible, and healthy, with the ability to lead an active life well into advanced age. Exercise should be an enjoyable lifetime habit.

9

Life is an obligation to endure. Endurance starts with the exercise of body, mind, and true essence, or spirit. The first step is to wake up and start working in your own lab, or yourself. Yourself is housed in, and around your physical body. So the first priority is to get your body in shape to attract and receive higher vibrations. We can initiate this by adhering to the proper requisites of good nutrition, spiritual enlivenment, and adequate physical exercise.

Most people on the planet, including children who live the lifestyle of the western world are grossly inactive and generally overweight. 21st century kids will spend much of their time playing computer games or watching television. And as people age, they tend to become even less active. The last 100 years has brought cars, elevators, golf carts, and now, even a vehicle (Segway) that walks for us. These things, and many others, contribute to less physical exertion.

But, there is one part of our body that most people exercise too much, and that is our jaw muscles. We eat too much. It is said that one pound of body fat contains enough energy for the average man to run 35 miles. This would equate to 8-10 hours of running. This caloric burn can be replaced in less than five minutes of eating. Your exercise program cannot compete with the mouth.

Health Benefits of Exercise

Direct physical activity in the form of exercise provides health, strength, power, endurance, flexibility, balance and agility, stress reduction, greater blood circulation, greater mobility, a stronger heart, stronger bones, joint lubrication, and other benefits, as well as a sense of well being.

Several other benefits of exercise: Less depression- Improved outlook on life- More self esteem- Prevents or reduces the severity of dementia and other neurological disorders- Increased ligament strength- Better sleep- Increased fat metabolism- Better carbohydrate metabolism- Increased fat loss- Quicker reflexes- Improved balance and coordination- Increased range of motion and strength- Fewer musculoskeletal injuries or problems- Quickens the absorption and expulsion of various growths and deposits- Increase in cardiac efficiency- Decrease in resting heart rate- Decrease in blood pressure- Stimulates bone growth- Increase in bone density- Improved posture- Increase in insulin sensitivity- Increase in high-density lipoprotein- Reduction in total cholesterol, and an increase in maximal oxygen uptake. It also improves the circulation of blood, lymph, and synovial fluid, the lubricating fluid made in joints, and these factors support the immune system. Quite an impressive list!

It also stimulates our white blood cells to produce a natural chemotherapy compound called interleukin 1. This in turn calls for the release of interleukin 2 that benefits the immune system. The detection and destruction of abnormal cells by various white blood cells and killer cells is increased by physical exercise. It increases by two times the blood plasma interferon levels that help fight cancer. And, muscle cells that are routinely put through their paces make more mitochondria. Mitochondria may be thought of as small internal factories that turn blood sugar into usable fuel. The more mitochondria, the more energy each cell will have at its beckon call. Regular exercise also prompts your body to sprout extra capillaries, the ultra-thin blood vessels that bring oxygen to cells. More blood, nutrients, and nerve energy are shuttled to areas of the body that are applied to action.

The whole anatomical body, including every cell, rebuilds itself completely every few years. It does this through our blood supply. Our blood carries destructive or creative properties to the rest of our body, depending on our lifestyle. The blood flowing through our body needs cleansing, and gets cleaned through the lymph system and the kidneys. The lymph system has no pump for movement as the blood has in the heart. Lymph fluid is dependent on muscle movement, especially the kind that increases the action of the lungs, diaphragm, and thorax, to move it through our system. Note: There is a simple exercise you can do that directly affects the lymph system. Stand with your feet shoulder width apart, arms to your side. Raise your arms in front of you, and pretend you are snow skiing.

So exercise plays a very important ongoing role in keeping our physiological processes operating properly. The health benefits of exercise can't, and must not be overlooked.

Get Going and Exercise

I have been an exercise aficionado all my life, and have had a great deal of experience in a wide array of regimens. These have included martial arts, weightlifting, power yoga, bicycling, volleyball, hiking, track and field, racquetball, horseback riding, baseball, basketball, and others. I always feel a continuous invigoration, and the different attacks on exercise seems to keep my body and mind rejuvenated, and adaptable to any situation that might come my way.

I recommend, as a basis for anyone that is not hampered in any way, to do some, weight resistance exercises, yoga, run, ride a bicycle, stretch, go swimming, do some abdominal and lower back strengthening, and any other type exercise you might enjoy. Participation in team sports is a lot of fun, in that it allows you to interact with others. Note: It doesn't matter how fit you are at any sport, when you start something new, you must start slow. You can't use new muscles in new ways and go full speed.

Many people get top heavy in one area of exercise, as they sometimes do with their eating habits. Women will just do aerobics, and men will just lift weights. The need is to utilize a variety of disciplines in your physical culture.

A well-rounded exercise program should be comprehensive enough to bring balance to your whole system, which includes mind and body. Awareness and physiology are closely related. **Intense aerobic exercises for your heart and lungs, weight resistance training for your musculature, skeleton and metabolism, and stretching should be mainstays of any program.**

13

People come home from work feeling tired, and thinking that they don't have the energy to workout, or they tend to think that it would make them even more tired. Fatigue toxins can build up and clog muscle tissue. Exercise helps get rid of these. Most people don't consider the fact that exercise should give you energy, not take it away. The fact of the matter is, that if they would catch a workout after the work hours, it would negate the lethargy associated with the day's work, and give them the energy to have a more alert and productive afternoon and evening.

Exercise should help keep us in a good frame of mind, keep us feeling light and energetic, improve our capacity for work, help us tolerate problems and difficulties more easily, help eliminate impurities, and stimulate our digestion. Also, sticking to your exercise program, and always completing the routines you set out to do is a good way to start establishing your word as law in your life.

Aerobic And Anaerobic Exercise

We know that oxygen plays a major role in everything that we do. Aerobic exercise causes you to take in oxygen, and is exercise performed over a certain amount of time. This type of exercise affects your lungs, heart, blood vessels, and respiratory muscles. Aerobic exercise, along with an appropriate diet, burns fat for fuel if done properly, and at the right time. It boosts your capacity to bring more oxygen to your organs and bodily systems.

Anaerobic exercises are those that require quick spurts of power or force, such as running speed sprints or weight resistance exercises. This type of exercise uses glycogen as its main fuel, and enables the body to store fat if improperly done.

Almost any kind of exercise can be aerobic or anaerobic, depending on how hard you push yourself. Important note: If you are not getting proper nutrition, and proper rest, and are exercising exclusively in an anaerobic fashion, your metabolism will burn glycogen as its main source of energy. And if your glycogen level starts to be depleted, your body will use blood sugar for an alternative fuel source, causing a drain on your health and energy.

Spend some time getting yourself aerobically fit before you try to add heavy weightlifting, or sports that call for explosive energy. Those weekend warriors who jump into an exercise or sport at a speed that causes them to create an anaerobic state very quickly are asking for trouble. You do not want to use up your oxygen when exercising. Your body may answer this call for a quick supply of blood by taking it from vital organs such as the kidneys or liver. This can cause these organs to lose a lot of oxygen, and can weaken them.

If you're way out of sorts, a brisk half hour walk

will help bring you back up to snuff. Walking is a very beneficial form of exercise for everyone. It necessitates the integration of our arms, legs and torso. Walking changes the pressure in body cavities due to skeletal motion rhythms and contractions, and relaxation of muscles. Daily walking at a good pace burns calories and increases enzyme and metabolic activity. Walking for only two miles can create caloric consumption for as long as twelve hours. Increased metabolism means that your body is helped to draw in nutrients from food and food supplements. It also increases your thirst, and that stimulates you to drink more water. Walking, with the exception of breathing is the most natural exercise the human does.

Yoga

As a form of exercise relative to overall health, yoga can be a good adjunct to a fitness lifestyle. Yoga is a mode of bodyweight exercise that can be added to your exercise program. It is ancient in age, and was scientifically developed by some of the most enlightened and knowledgeable minds of antiquity to balance the different limbs in relationship to the whole body in harmonic proportion. This correlates the magnetic resonance of the motive apparatus of the body with its internal organs, and more importantly, its glandular and nervous system, which ties into the inner bodies through the nadis and chakra systems described in **Life is a Science, Not a Roll of the Dice** and **Infinity of Intrigue (amazon.com).** Other forms of exercise used excessively misalign the bodily structure.

Just as the earth has its axis, so does man. Our spinal column plays an all-important role in our functions, and controls balance in our movements. Whether you lift weights, attend aerobics classes, run, participate in the various sports, or whatever, you will create tightness or disproportionate stresses on your frame, and especially the spinal column. Yoga, on the other hand, by nature of its synergistic design, strengthens, balances, straightens out, loosens up, and aligns your physicality. Yoga, over a period of time, will align what has become unaligned from the over use of other types of exercise. Most people, including myself, employ and enjoy other modes of exercise and sports, because they all have benefits when used in proper context. However, yoga sun salutations 1&2 in themselves, when combined and sequenced, and done for fifteen or twenty minutes nonstop is a good, quick workout. They work and stretch all your muscles at the same time. They are convenient and effective as a warm-up exercise and a cool-down exercise. They can help level out imbalances you may have in your body's alignment. The sun salutations help put blood and oxygen into muscles, and help alleviate any muscle soreness or stiffness from over-exercising by flushing out excess lactic acid from muscles. They help train your muscles to work collectively due to the angles the postures produce, and they add to muscle stamina. See the book **Yoga Compact (amazon.com)** for illustrated sun salutations and a great on-the-go workout.

Note on osteoporosis: A decade or more after maturity, blood supply to our spinal disks becomes scarcer. From this point on, physical movement provides nourishment for the spine. Manipulation of the spine through lengthening and stretching draws the necessary fluids in and out of the spinal disks. People become shorter, and lose flexibility as they age because of gradual shrinkage of the disks. Certain movements, especially yoga exercises, help to maintain space between the vertebrae and enable a person to maintain flexibility and balance into advanced age.

It can be a good companion to other programs or sports. It teaches one focus and discipline, along with its physical health building qualities. Through continual practice, yoga trains the mind and builds concentration. It is a very sophisticated form of physical therapy.

A certain form of yoga called *power yoga* is one of the most well rounded, and thorough forms of yoga that exists. It creates strength, endurance, and flexibility. This form ties the various movements together in an uninterrupted flow. This flow is also at the same time tied to the constant flow of breath. These two factors, along with the bearing of your own bodyweight, and the flexing and tensing aspects, operate together to produce tremendous heat, which loosens up everything from muscles to joints. It aligns what is misaligned by working on the spine and other areas. The heat produced makes the tendons, joints, and muscles more supple and amenable to being properly reshaped. Ancient *astanga yoga*, now called *power yoga*, is the Cadillac of yoga exercise, and is also a highly effective form of meditation when done properly.

Just as other forms of exercise may not be suited for everyone due to particular limitation, so is the case with power yoga. When pursued to its fullest extent, it is very intricate and time consuming. It takes a tremendous amount of dedication to complete its major segments, and an intense tenacity to continue day in and day out. I speak from experience. The average person won't develop and sustain the constant focus needed to make this habitual. However, if you can break the law of averages, and are so inclined, it is one of the ultimate yoga practices at this point in time.

Note: Through research and experience, I do not recommend yoga as a stand-a-lone exercise regimen. In its general application, it lacks certain strength and conditioning factors, and can be problematic for some individuals relative to certain postures and stretching factors. However, it can be of great value, especially sun salutations I&I, when used in conjunction with an overall exercise program.

The Warm-Up and Cool Down

Pay attention to this! A warm-up period of 5-10 minutes is recommended before resistance exercise or high intensity aerobic exercise. It causes the fatty acids in your body to get into your bloodstream. This helps to ensure that your body is burning fat rather than blood sugar. If you skip the warm up and jump into your routine, even if it is aerobic, you will hamper fat burning. It also enables your body to slowly and intelligently distribute blood to the places that need it, as opposed to taking it from some of the critical organs, as we have mentioned. It increases blood flow to muscles by over 50%, which gives better muscle contraction, starts sweating earlier to regulate body temperature which promotes faster neurotransmitter connection, and activates the carb/fat metabolism hormones. Walking, jogging in place, or doing jumping jacks is suitable, however, the Sun Salutations are ideal. They provide a movement and a rest to the muscles, and a range of motion that loosens the joints and connective tissue.

The cool down is equally important! Always allow yourself a cool down period of 5-10 minutes. This will allow your blood to be cleaned, redistributed, and re-oxygenated. If you do not cool down properly, your blood can settle or pool in your muscles. A common practice is to walk.

Aerobic Exercise: Right Way & Wrong Way

Aerobic exercise is geared to exercise lungs, and is necessary and beneficial for their maximum efficiency. It is also beneficial for the heart when done properly. The various aerobic exercises can include running, bicycling, swimming, yoga, cross-country skiing, rowing, jumping rope, and others. Weightlifting and bodyweight exercise also offers a certain amount of aerobic conditioning. Note: If you always run, or train on a bike, the changes and effects will be mostly confined to your lower body. A more effective workout would be to use whole-body aerobic exercises such as cross-country skiing, swimming, rowing, or power yoga. These types of aerobics burn fat more efficiently throughout your entire body due to the fact that they bring more muscle mass into play, which in turn will cause more oxygen consumption and a heavier expenditure of calories.

The main objective of aerobics is to expend enough energy to force your lungs to take more oxygen into your system, so make sure to breathe as much as you can while doing aerobic work. Breathing, in and of itself is a form of aerobic exercise, and setting aside a few minutes of deep breathing before and after any exercise regimen will be very beneficial. Also, any time you think about it during the day, take in some deep breaths.

Certain types of aerobic exercise are a waste of time, and can wreak havoc with your health, and may even kill you. People that lived many ages before us did not run, jump, and gyrate for an hour at a time several times a week. Most likely, they ran all out to catch some prey, or to get away from danger. And they probably did a lot of walking here and there.

The modern world does not represent the

environment that our bodies are currently designed for. Our genes, and our bodily structure are still basically the same as eons ago. The conditions of the world have outpaced our adaptation to it. Physical exploits needed in the olden times to live and survive have gone by the wayside. As a result, muscular and lean have morphed into flabby, weak, and sickly.

As you age, the ability to keep disease at bay and hold on to strength and stamina is lessened due to the fact that your lungs start to shrink; the lung cells can't be replaced at the die-off rate. The smaller they become negotiates an earlier death. It is said that at age 50 lung power is decreased by 40%, and by 80, 60%. But, if you have been acutely out of shape, these averages may be increased, even to the point that, at 80, you may have lost 90%. Aging is not the only factor relative to lungpower. Being obese lowers it significantly. A weight-laden chest restricts lung operation and increases aging and age related diseases. A doctor can test the lungs using a pulmonary function test.

Activity that causes an oxygen debt is the key to better lung function. This is getting to the stage of exertion when the lungs want more oxygen than they can get. The need is to go beyond the comfortable activity zone or the so-called 'aerobic zone' and get to an oxygen depletion state in a quick manner. Running wind sprints is an example of high exertion exercise that will get you there fast. Shortness of breath will occur as soon as you stop, and you will be panting to quickly get oxygen. By periodically giving your body an oxygen debt, you force it to adapt to a greater lung capacity. Remember that lung capacity decreases, as you get older. The standard medium forms of lung-involved exercise won't do the trick because they don't force the lungs to ramp up their function. Without this continual ramping up of lungpower, the lungs stay in a mode of decline. Your heart attack risk can also rise substantially.

Extended duration and less intense exercise such as standard cardio, jogging, aerobics class, bike riding, and long distance running have an adverse effect on the body. Your heart and lungs will actually decrease in size to conserve energy and function more efficiently at a lower level of effort. Distance runners are more susceptible to heart attack, joint stress injury, and bone and cartilage damage, along with artery hardening, to name a few. Extended session exercise produces continual stress on the heart, and allows no time for intermittent recovery. The heart and blood vessels may become chronically inflamed, along with muscle wastage, and bone loss. And science has shown that inflammation, not cholesterol, triggers heart disease.

Also, don't do intense aerobic exercise for an hour at a time several days a week. Intense, steady state aerobics will produce a depressed metabolic rate. The muscle wasting produced by high intensity, steady state action, causes this. This wasting can also signify other muscle and health related compromises. This type of body locomotion is said to cause elevated cortisol production, oxidative stress, excessive muscular fatigue, decreases testosterone and HGH levels, increases appetite, causes continued stress to feet, ankles, and knees, wastes too much time to burn a few calories, leads to the loss of fast twitch muscle fibers, creates muscular imbalance, and inflexibility, causes adrenal burnout, and more. Doing excessive cardio aerobics, and not utilizing a high degree of antioxidant protection will also cause skin damage akin to that caused by cigarette smoking.

Steady, low intensity aerobic exercise is not the

best method, but, as opposed to the high intensity routines performed in some classes, it would be better health-wise. When you exercise too hard, many times your muscles can't get enough stored fat from your fat tissue (adipose), so they switch to another energy source. They look to the carbohydrate that is stored within the muscle tissue itself.

It can be mentioned that steady state exercise used by long distance runners makes them susceptible to infections and serious diseases, such as heart disease. This type of exercise does not train, or allow, the heart to recover, as intervals of intense exertion with an in-between recovery period allows.

Cardio is the term generally used for conditioning/strengthening the heart. However, as generally done, it does not make the heart stronger, because strength and endurance are produced by different exercises. Cardio, as in exercising for an extended period of time, doesn't produce what the heart needs. It can actually reduce the heart's ability to respond to certain situations. To lower the risk of heart disease, exercise that is intense is needed, not a lengthy endurance mode. Short interval exercise performed at a high intensity level is actually safer, and necessarily, gives your heart and lungs reserve power that can serve you well when there is a sudden demand for physical action. Intense interval training with a progression in intensity gets the job done. You are able to react and adapt more readily to any situation that may pop up. If you want to have a strong heart, a lean muscular body, and plenty of lungpower, don't do general aerobics. BTW, who looks more healthy and fit, sprinters or runners? No contest; sprinters.

Experimenting with all the exercise video-frap marketed, along with the expense and wasted time involved does not work, and is ludicrous. The dancing, kicking, punching, jumping, and bouncing around for an hour video routines are an unnecessary waste of time. Your body is not built to thrive on this type of medium exertion exercise.

A twenty-minute session divided into short intervals of intense bursts of physical effort, followed by resting to recover is the way to go. This type exercise lends to increased lung volume, reserve capacity for the heart, faster fat loss, an increased metabolism, increased insulin sensitivity, strong bones, muscle growth, enhanced sexual performance, a stronger immune system and charged-up energy.

Short, intense exertion intervals followed by a rest signals your lungs to expand. By consistently using and upping your exertion techniques over time, adapting to this type exercise increases the lung's volume and power. The good results are many, to include: healthier organs, increased blood circulation, reduced inflammation that may lead to heart attack or stroke, increased stamina, and other benefits I won't list. Even individuals with emphysema or COPD can improve their lot by this method. It is quite possible to be 70 years old and have the lungpower of the average 30 year old!

A 20-minute session, divided into short, intense intervals is the way to go. It is simply going as hard as you can until you have to stop, and then resting until your breathing returns to normal. And then you go again. You repeat these high intensity intervals until you have used up twenty minutes. Do a five-minute warm-up and then do your first high intensity interval. Begin timing your session at the start of the first interval, and end the session in the neighborhood of twenty minutes.

Start out at the level you can handle. Depending on your condition, some people may have to walk their interval, then jog, and then run. The goal is to work up to your max output relative to your ability. You can run, bike, jump rope, swim, or whatever for your interval training.

It is said that the heart's output and blood to the lungs may increase by over 400%, and almost two times the amount of oxygen and blood is received by the brain using this methodology, as compared to results gotten from the effort put forth in medium exertion exercise like cardio/aerobics or endurance training. This is a hell of a difference in value received and time spent!

The Metabolic Equivalent (MET) is the amount of oxygen used by a normal, seated, person. Mets increase with the intensity of exercise. Walking at four mph produces 5 mets, and jogging at six mph produces 8 mets. A high peak exercise capacity, such as high intensity interval sprints, not only causes the intake of fresh oxygen, but it also burns up a greater amount of oxygen than your normal exercise exertion factor. It consists of getting to the point of having to catch your breath.

This aspect of exercise has been shown to be a better qualifier of how long we can live than the factors of high blood pressure, cholesterol, diabetes, smoking, and even heart disease. Your chance of living longer goes up with an increase in your mets. So, if you want to live longer, increase your peak exercise capacity.

Exercise should help in the loss of fat, not muscle. Aerobics, as we apply nowadays does just the opposite. The aspect of fat control through raising the metabolic rate depends much on muscle strength and size, not aerobics. The aerobics craze that has engulfed us in the last few decades is unnecessary and not as beneficial to your health as its proponents would have you believe.

Short, high intensity aerobic spurts will burn a

certain amount of fat, and the burning of calories overall is much greater using this type activity, as opposed to steady state only. Also, the time following your workout will also burn more calories and fat. And the intensity will produce a higher level of fitness and health.

For your aerobic training, the high intensity interval session is the way to go for lung and heart health, fat loss without muscle loss, overall aerobic conditioning, and time efficiency. Note: It is THE exercise to activate the super fast muscle fibers.

Short High Intensity Exercise for Fat Loss

Let me continue on by adding to the last above paragraphs. You may have heard about the idea that you have to perform exercise for 15 or 20 minutes so you can get to the so-called 'fat burning zone." This may seem logical, but it is false.

The body burns carbohydrate such as glycogen, fat, or protein for energy. The intensity and time length of certain exercise will determine the quantity of energy derived from one of these sources.

The body uses something named ATP for the first 2 or 3 minutes, as it is the most available energy at your disposal. After this short time period, the body changes over to carbohydrate stores in the muscle tissue for energy. After around 20 minutes, the body switches to fat for energy.

Here is what you need to understand. Exercise that is low in intensity, such as walking a good distance, gets a great amount of energy from carbs, but just around 15-18% from fat. Now, if you up your exercise intensity to medium, like jogging, running, bike riding, etc, or other extended duration exercise, fat will supply around 50+% of the energy. However, if you jump to high intensity exercise, most of your energy will come from carbs, not fat. So, the propensity for people that want to lose fat is to do medium intensity exercise because it shows that this type burns more fat <u>during</u> a session. But, this is misleading, if you want to lose fat. Why? The body, when burning fat during a medium exercise session, senses a need to produce more fat for future medium intensity, extended duration exercise sessions. This type exercise can cause you to give up muscle, even organ tissue, and preserve fat.

What you need to know is this. What happens with the body after exercise is more important than what happens during an exercise session. When you do short spurts of high intensity exercise over a time period of 20 minutes or less, the body does not get the 'store fat as energy' message because you're not exercising long enough to use the low-release energy fat for fuel. Instead, the body will use high-octane carbs in muscle for energy. Then, after the workout, the body will drop back and use slow burning fat. This fat burning may last up to 48 hours, and this means you actually burn several times more fat than using traditional, medium extended duration exercise that burns a little fat during the session, but actually causes the body to produce and store more fat after the session.

So, you want to do high intensity exercise interval sessions that last no longer that 20 minutes, so you won't burn fat during the session, but will get the fat burning effect long after the session is over, along with the many benefits associated with this type exercise, as discussed previously in the material.

Resistance Exercise

Most people today think that the heart is the main cog that physical health revolves around, and that an inordinate amount of aerobic exercise is needed to exercise the heart muscle. But the heart, as a muscle, does not have a great dependency on aerobic exercise. It gets plenty of action by performing its constant duty unless you are extremely lethargic. Exercising the muscles that surround the heart will benefit the health of the heart. Metabolically speaking, the muscles are of greater interest than the heart. The metabolic focus of the body is the skeletal muscles. They contain the greatest amount of mitochondria, the most water, the most ongoing chemistry, the greatness heat production, and the largest blood supply.

An age related condition known as *sarcopenia* slows metabolism and causes the common loss of muscle usually found in people over the age of forty or fifty. It leads to bone loss, and as much as five to seven pounds of muscle tissue each decade.

The skeleton, being your base structure, should receive attention. When we use our muscles in resistance activities, it transmits bioelectrical and mechanical signals that create greater bone density.

Note. The reduced metabolic rate and the recession of caloric intake as we age is not a part of aging as some would have us believe. It is a result of the lesser amount of muscle due to becoming more sedentary. Muscle is active tissue that demands nourishment. Fat is passive. It resides as a storage form of body energy.

General athletic decline starts as early as age twenty, and assumes a downhill pace dictated to a great degree by your exercise habits. The average person who reaches the age of fifty, and has not done resistance training for the past thirty years will lose from ten to fifteen pounds of muscle mass, and will have replaced this muscle with ten to fifteen pounds of fat. This person will be carrying around more fat weight with less muscle to move it. This puts more of a strain on his energy pool and his heart. When we move into middle age, we can't eat as much as we did in the past without gaining weight because our metabolism slows and burns hundreds of calories less each day. By the time an individual reaches the age of seventy, he, or she, may lose as much as forty percent of their muscle and strength. The most helpful antidote for this is weight resistance exercise.

Resistance exercise builds a leaner, more muscular physique. Your metabolism won't be elevated for very long after an aerobic workout. But even at rest, an additional thirty to fifty calories a day will be burned for every pound of muscle you gain. If you want to boost your metabolic rate even more, utilize what are called multi-joint compound exercises such as pull-ups, push-ups, squats, and dead lifts. This type works several muscle groups at once, and is the 'meat and potatoes' of an exercise regimen. This format will also enable you to handle poundage that will bring greater changes in size and strength.

These compound exercises performed with serious intensity are said to increase the circulation of growth hormone and testosterone, which are noted for their muscle building properties. These hormones also assist in the breaking down of fat in the body. After you get yourself stronger and more in shape, you might want to do some isolation exercises to bring out the definition of various body parts. These are exercises that concentrate on specific body parts such as shoulders, arms, calves, etc.

Note: The middle age concerns of losing muscle, lower energy levels, skin wrinkling, excess weight gain, decreased bone density, increased body fat, and slower metabolism is directly related to the decline of growth hormone (HGH). This comes with the aging process. HGH can slow the aging process, help get rid of body fat, and upgrade your musculature quality to a great degree.

It has been demonstrated that returning growth hormone to your system brings back the vitality of a younger age, and holds back the hands of time. As a result, there has been a great interest in restoring growth hormone. All sorts of pills have appeared, along with expensive injections. And, as usual, along with the magic bullet comes problems. Stay away from these approaches, unless you have a medical condition in which your physician prescribes them.

There is a proven and safe way to activate growth hormone. Aggressive anaerobic exercise using short, intense bursts of speed in segments, or increments, can increase HGH growth hormone by as much as 500%! Keeping the cells permeable to receive the growth hormone by controlling your blood sugar is very important. This type exercise does this.

It is important to exercise the three types of muscle fiber in our muscle composition. The three types are super fast, fast, and slow twitch. On average, we have 60% fast, which includes super fast, and 40% slow twitch fibers. The fast twitch fiber (IIa) moves 5X faster than the slow twitch (I). The super-fast (IIx) is 10x faster than the slow twitch fibers. Each person's fiber composition can vary somewhat due to genetics, etc.

The way our muscles are trained determines development. Track sprinters who train with more intense bursts of speed have a higher percentage of the super-fast, while endurance training produces a slower twitch muscle.

Generally, 95% of people, after the age of eighteen, and I'm only talking about people who continue to exercise after high school, start and remain slow twitch exercisers. So, the majority of people are on a downhill run with growth hormone as a result of this. The aging process speeds up, energy levels go down, weight goes up, various diseases have more opportunity to gain a foothold, and muscle strength and tone go down.

So, even though a few people continue a program of weight resistance and cardio, they are not producing HGH because they are only exercising slow twitch muscles. The other half of their musculature, the fast and super fast twitch fibers, are not worked because of not doing high intensity type exercise. Therefore, half of our muscles begin to atrophy at a young age. This is the reason we can't jump into high-intensity anaerobic sessions. The muscle fiber needed for this type exercise has atrophied, and has to be brought back slowly using proper methods.

You may have heard that exercise itself causes free radicals. This is true, but only in small amounts, if not exacerbated by over training. In fact, the free radicals produced during proper training actually benefit the heart by providing oxidant defenses into the heart muscle.

High intensity exercise that produces lactic acid is thought to have antioxidant capabilities. If you intersperse segments of exercise that will bring you to a momentary state of being out of breath, the body will call for the blood system to bring in (scavenge) all the oxygen it can to repay the oxygen debt. It searches for whatever can be oxidized. This is one of the reasons that you feel so good after an intense session. An example would be to move quickly, take very little rest, between the sets of your resistance exercise, whether it is lifting weights, using cable bands, or bodyweight exercises, and using the high intensity aerobic type sprints.

Also, inserting these intervals of high intensity will elevate the amount of calories burned during your workout, and your post exercise fat burning may last as much as forty-eight hours.

One pound of muscle burns around seventy-five calories a day, but fat burns only two or three. An hour of general aerobic exercise will burn more calories than an hour of strength promoting exercise, but the strength training will keep on working for you throughout the day, whereas general aerobics will only burn calories during the aerobic exercise period. For every ten pounds of muscle mass you gain you will burn an extra 500 to 750 calories per day. That is four to five thousand calories a week!

Note: If you participate in athletic competition, know that fat and protein increases athletic performance better than "carb-loading." The burning of fat as fuel enables you to exercise harder and longer. And you use less oxygen, so you breathe less, and decrease oxidative stress relative to aging. More oxygen is required to burn by sugar, and this may even harm tissues while exercising.

Insulin tells your body to store energy, not burn it. To burn fat, athletes should train using low carb diets. However, in order to increase your glycogen stores, it is sometimes feasible to eat a carb meal the night before participating in a strenuous sports event.

Note. Resistance training for insulin resistance is more efficient than aerobic exercise. Resistance training will increase the insulin sensitivity of your muscles. It also increases blood flow to the muscles.

Note. Find out if you are overweight by checking out your BMI. This is body mass index. Here is the formula. 1. Figure out how many inches tall you are. For an example, let's assume you are a woman 5 ft. tall, or 60 inches. 2. Multiply that figure by itself. 60x60=3600. 3. Divide your wt. by the figure in step 2. If you weigh 120 lbs. you would divide 120 by 3600. Round the result off to the nearest decimal point. 4. Multiply the result by 703. The result is your BMI. The World Health Organization defines overweight as a score of 25 or more, and obesity as 30 or more. Races of different body types can vary by a couple of points.

Attention ladies: Many women are concerned that resistance exercises will make them took like professional bodybuilding specimens. This won't happen unless you are going to spend four to five hours a day at the gym, and at the same time consume the diet of these particular types. Most women are after the effect of body sculpting for normal muscular definition and curves. Women talk about shaping-up. This means that the body should be firm, the waistline, the thighs, and the buttocks should be tight, and their size minimized as much as nature and genetics will allow, and that the whole body will present a shapely muscular definition. These particular qualities can only be sufficiently produced by resistance exercises. Aerobic exercises do not shape the body.

Here, let me note the word *symmetry*. It denotes an evolutionary hint to health. And researchers know that tumors and pathologies create distorted asymmetries.

Genetically, men have more muscle mass than women. Due to this, the metabolic rate of men is somewhere around fifteen percent higher than women. This, along with their higher testosterone level makes men naturally leaner, and gives them a slight advantage in muscle building. Women have more body fat in the hips, thighs, and waist than men as a result of these factors. But with a little effort, women can overcome these disadvantages.

The primary reason for exercise is to renew or improve the functional ability to control our body. The most natural and practical forms of resistance exercise are body weight exercises. They use your own body weight. This has been the basic mode for warriors and physical exhibitionists, such as strongmen, for innumerable ages. The degree to which you can handle your body weight will greatly determine the physical shape you are in. The technical term for these exercises is *somatatrophic*. They include such forms as leg squats using just your bodyweight, push ups, pull ups (chins), dips, sit ups, etc. Exercises relative to these are called *asomatatrophic*, and would include weightlifting and certain sports.

For your body to have proper and efficient movement, the muscles must work together in coordination. Body weight exercises, along with power yoga, free weight exercises and cable band exercises achieve this better than other modes of resistance training due to the fact that they force your stabilizer muscles to come into action in a much more pronounced way. We can look at the bench press to see this. A bench press performed on a machine apparatus promotes linear strength and does away with stabilization. Standard bench-presses with a barbell or cable calls not only for force to push the bar or cable up, but also for a stabilizing effort to keep the bar from leaning side to side. The common push up also calls for stabilization as a factor. Free weight and cable exercises make you use your own center of gravity and forces the co-condition of the stabilizer, neutralizer and postural muscles called into play with a given exercise.

If you are a young person, and have a desire or

calling to be a serious power lifter or bodybuilder, stick top heavy with multi-joint compound exercises to build size and strength. After you've gotten into a higher state of shape and strength, then work in the isolation exercises for defining specific body parts. Note: These two classes that display brute strength or cosmetic appearances do not produce an all round functional athletic ability. They also put extra stress and strain on your bodily systems, especially if you are approaching middle age.

As you can readily observe, most of the people pictured in the muscle periodicals are at one end of the spectrum when it comes to what most people want to do with their bodies. People wrongly equate tightness with strength. Severe tightness over a period of time will actually diminish strength. If you constantly overdo weightlifting, you can reduce mobility along with strength due to the fact that your muscles are held in a condition of partial contraction. This can tire them out.

Note to heavy lifters: Lifting heavy weights continually to the point of failure or exhaustion is unnatural and harmful. Using your own body weight to produce muscularity and maintain it best suits the human body. This uses the body's natural function, and is the safe and best way to strengthen tendons and ligaments. Extreme muscle pumping over a period of time can actually lead to muscle exhaustion and other physiological problems.

To offset the momentary effects, and possible long-term negative effects of continual heavy lifting, be sure to do a brief, low intensity cool down. This will help in keeping your cardiovascular system healthy. It will give the heart a chance to operate against a low perfusion pressure, and help venous return.

Bulking up, and lifting heavy over the long haul won't allow you to function or feel as well as you should. Your speed and flexibility is generally sacrificed to a degree. But the integration of body weight exercises, power yoga and cable band routines will produce muscles that feel different, and better. And they will act different. You will feel more capable in all areas, and be ready to jump over tall buildings. And, you will discover that you are faster and more efficient at whatever you attempt to do. Also, as we get older, the stress and strain of very heavy lifting can cause, or exacerbate, excessive free radical damage, along with other problems.

There is less potential damage in all things when you lean toward the side of moderation, as opposed to excess. Over-exercising in any mode can be inflammatory to the body.

If you are hell-bent on traditional bodybuilding, you can find useful information about proper form, along with routines that will be suited for your particular needs at the local gym, and in the many muscle and health magazines and websites. Most of these offer pictures of specific exercises and proper form along with up to the minute data, not only on the latest modes in the physical culture department, but also keep current on cutting edge information and products relating to internal health as well. But don't get unduly influenced by their nutritional or supplement advertising.

I will mention one product that many health authorities suggest in supplement form. It is creatine. It is said to promote muscle growth even without exercise. But, it works better if you do. It is also said to bolster your recuperative powers relative to injuries, and even illness. And it improves heart function. Do your research before taking creatine.

Note: Some sources suggest that the traditional bodybuilding parameters of eight to twelve reps with a sixty second rest period used in sets overly stresses the muscular system, especially when using machines. Know that the nervous system controls the muscular system, and that both have a relative relationship. To improve the functioning of your nervous system, perform your exercises at progressively higher speeds.

Also, try tensing, or contracting the other muscles of your body during each particular set of resistance exercise and you will experience an automatic increase in the intensity of the contraction of the target muscles. Squeezing the bar during the bench press can increase the poundage you are able to handle.

It is important to know that the largest scope and longest sustained biological improvements of exercise in health are accomplished with strength training. These improvements include cosmetics, and also strength and endurance, joint stability, metabolic rate, bone density, and vascular efficiency.

Super Slow Resistance Training: This is going super slow in an individual weightlifting set, along with working the targeted muscle, or muscle group, to exhaustion. The slow speed is said to take out the momentum aspect of a lift and bring more muscle fibers into play. Said to minimize joint stress. The idea is to perform one set of a particular exercise super slow to failure. This crowd works out for thirty minutes, once or twice a week. The idea is that a super intense workout necessitates a recuperation period of anywhere from five to seven days to produce optimal benefit.

Note: A general rule of thumb for lifting weights (not super slow), such as in a biceps curl, would be to use a count of 1-2 on the up, and 1-2-3-4 on the down, or negative aspect. The negative aspect is very important in weightlifting. In super slow, you could use a 10 count up and 10 down.

Super slow training has become a method of choice for some police, certain Special Forces groups, paramilitary groups, and others. It takes patience and concentration. It can cut the time of your weight routine by 70%. It can be used in body weight exercises as well as free weight exercises.

There are a number of intelligent and highly credible super slow physical culturists who are trying to bring this modality to the forefront of the exercise scene presently ensconced in our society. And there are gyms with equipment designed for super slow that are springing up all around the country. To read more about this type weight training, view the *Super Slow Exercise Guild* web site. However, it should be noted that many exercise experts say that to train slow is to be slow.

Pushing, Pulling, Or Pumping Rubber: This is using cable bands for your resistance exercises. Many noted physical culturists find that this method is superior to pumping iron for overall functional fitness, both aerobically, and anaerobically. I have read that the cable idea, or strand, came from the bowman of yore. Pulling the bow back required a certain amount of strength, along with centering your balance and steadiness. The stronger the pound pull of the bow, the further the arrow would fly, and the deeper the penetration. An anemic and weak individual could not utilize the strong bow.

Using cables is like muscle going against muscle. It can seem like a competition. You can do more exercises, use more angles, have a wider range of motion, and it offers more pushing and pulling movements than conventional weights or machines.

I have been using cables as an adjunct to my other modes of exercise for a long time. There is no comparison, as far as I am concerned, as to their efficiency as opposed to pumping iron. Better results are produced in many aspects. The number of movements and angles available is fantastic. And there is convenience and time saved by not having to go to the gym, or mess with the different machines, weights, and other contraptions, not to mention waiting around for your turn to use all these things. The results and the feel you can get from cable routines will astound you.

Let me emphasize some other information. To have power, you must have alignment and balance. Alignment between the upper and lower body is necessary, and comes from training the core areas such as the musculature of the spine, the abdominal area, the pelvic region and the shoulder blades. To fully acquire power and stability in these areas, they should be trained in as many positions and angles (frontal, lateral, diagonal and rotational) as possible.

Most weight machine designs do not allow stability training. They are generally geared toward muscle isolation and don't let your muscles work together as the human body design dictates. Bodyweight exercises, cables, and power yoga strengthen and integrate muscle connections. One reason is that they include the core areas in the movement. Bodyweight exercises make you work harder by bringing more musculature into play, and this causes you to burn more calories by increasing metabolism. It also forces you to bring in more oxygen that creates more body heat and energy.

There are many muscles on the body that are not brought into play sufficiently, or at all, by pumping iron. These muscles can be reached by using a combination of the modes just mentioned. You'll find muscles you didn't know you had. And you can create a body that looks better and manlier than the 'bodybuilder' look.

Most of the things we do in life, including athletics,

use the whole body, legs, back, abs, and so forth. It is prudent to train your muscles in the ways that cause you to balance, and use overall strength and power. Most of the sports athletes that are lean, strong, quick and powerful are not using bodybuilding routines to get that way. They workout by practicing their sport, and if they are smart, by integrating bodyweight exercises, cables, and power yoga into the mix.

STRETCHING and FLEXIBILITY

This is also very important to your fitness and health level. As you age, stretching becomes more necessary because your connective tissue becomes increasingly more brittle over time. Stretching to become more flexible means to work the muscle.

Doing special flexibility programs for dancers, certain programs for gymnasts, martial arts, and others are not good for the average person when done in extended sessions over a long period of time. They are especially not good for properly acquired strength, or for joint mobility. Most retired dancers and gymnasts have severe problems. Doing daily martial arts workouts for years produced problems with my knees and arms. I have since overcome these problems with diet, and by a greater focus on strength work and power yoga.

Permanently stretched ligaments, and the other problems that many popular programs produce are not brought to the attention of the fitness consumer. Tendons have very little elastic property. They are basically static, and not subject to being stretched. The hyper-mobility syndrome that arises from these programs cause pain, balance instability, and dysfunction. Overly limber and loose joints lean toward being unstable and are more subject to injury.

The contractile element in the belly region of a muscle is very elastic. Knowing this, it is logical that the more you can contract it, the more you can stretch it. Muscles put through a full range of motion can remain flexible for life.

Relative to this, here is some interesting information about John Grimek. He was a famous, large and very muscular specimen. It is noted that he ended his 1940 Mr. America posing routine by landing in a full split, and then when he stood to bow to the audience, he placed his elbows on the floor with his knees straight.

Weight resistance does not make muscles inflexible. The idea of becoming muscle bound arises from the strongmen of old who were very fat. They were actually fat bound. Healthy and normal flexibility is a by-product of proper weightlifting. In truth, stronger muscles are more flexible.

We need greater strength, not more flexibility. Note to women: Due to female hormones, and their childbearing ability, women are already hyper-mobile, and too flexible in some respects. Over increasing their flexibility makes for joint instability, and renders them more susceptible and prone to injury. Women need to acquire greater muscular strength to protect their joints. And weight resistance is the only way to shape and firm the feminine physique.

So, muscularity breeds flexibility. Trying to gain over-flexibility by these other means can damage the structural integrity of joints. The steady stress and strain on tendons and ligaments from some other forms of exercise is harmful. The belly of the muscle is the only thing that can be effectively stretched, and that is accomplished by contraction. Stretching is important in that it elongates the protective sheath of connective tissue (fascia) covering muscles and muscle cells. Muscle gets more room to grow when this fascia is stretched. Stretching lends to greater muscle shape, improves muscle separation, and can even improve bone structure.

When you stretch a muscle far enough it will cause a reflex, which will make it contract. Continued repetition of the stretching, slowly allows you to postpone this response through small measured advances, and results in an increase in your range of motion.

Also, if you train heavy with weights, it can be helpful to stretch to offset the effects, which may include a temporary lower range of motion, and even injury. Stretching also seems to have a positive effect on strength gains. Yoga sun salutations I & II are good stretch routines. You can do them before, and after your weight workout. More than any other warm-up, they cause an action/rest combination to the muscles, and offer a range of motion that loosens the joints and connective tissue. If you use the standard stretch practices of traditional exercisers, you should stretch after your regular exercise session. At that time the body is warm, and the connective tissue is more elastic.

Normal stretching enables muscles to fire more efficiently, and to not shut down as a response to stretched tendons. The so-called golgi tendon organs are situated in the tendons near the ends of the muscle fibers. These golgi tendons act as stretch receptors, and react to changes in muscle or tendon length as a muscle or tendon is stretched or contracts in a strong manner, thereby acting as a safety mechanism. It is thought that when an action passes a certain critical point, a quick reflex acts to stop the over contraction or stretch. The muscle quickly relaxes, the over tension is alleviated, and possible injury may be avoided.

When you fail doing a max rep in weight lifting, it is not only because of muscle fatigue; it is also due to the golgi tendon organs being activated and shutting down your muscle activity. It is possible to raise this threshold by stretching muscles and ligaments on a regular basis, and realize a fifteen to twenty percent gain in muscle strength.

Righting and Tilting Reflex Exercises

As we grow older, we tend to lose these reflexes to a degree. An example of righting, which is walking on a fixed object, would be walking on a balance beam. If you have access to railroad tracks, you might want to go for a walk on them every so often, or something of a similar nature. An example of tilting, which happens when an object under you moves, would be surfing. If you don't live near the ocean, you can ride a bicycle, or go to the mall and ride the escalator. And, if you're a serious tilting aficionado, you might want go to a country-western club and ride the mechanical bull! A Swiss Ball is a good exercise prop for both these reflexes.

Relaxation Exercise

This will top off a session very nicely. It will release tension and give you a good feeling all over. Lie flat on your back with your arms on the floor, palms up. Tense each listed body part for a count of ten, then relax the body part for a count of ten. Breathe deeply throughout each segment.

The order: Toes > Ankles > Calves > Thighs > Suck in Anus and hold, then relax. Butt Muscles > Lower Back > Abdominals > Upper Back and Shoulders > Chest > Triceps > Biceps > Forearms > Hands > Stick Tongue out of mouth, then relax it > Neck-Face (You figure it out) > Finish. Lie still;

breathe slowly and naturally for eight breaths.

Note: A body massage is great for relaxation. It also helps improve the function of the circulatory, lymphatic, and nervous system.

Breath Importance and Breath Exercise

Breathing, as we have noted, is an exercise within itself. Don't neglect it, because it is a most important factor. When it comes to weightlifting, breathe out on the exertion part, and in on the negative part of the exercise, unless otherwise directed. In other forms of exercise, let your lungs set the pace as they necessarily see fit to do. Steady breathing will enable you to work out longer and harder. Tidbit: At the base of the brain is a nerve center that is very sensitive to the amount of carbon dioxide that is in the blood. When there is more carbon dioxide in the blood than is acceptable, the nerve center sends out nerve signals to the chest muscles to increase your rate of breath, thereby bringing in more oxygen.

Breath exercises have many benefits, especially when you breathe mindfully (paying attention to your breath), and this can modify and quicken your 'in house' self-regulating physiological and bio-energetic mechanisms. By proper body oxygenation you are aligning your internal and energetic balance, and this has a definite effect on your nervous system. Collectively, all this affects the whole body, even down to the cellular level, including your subtle energy systems, as described in **Life is a Science, Not a Roll of the Dice (amazon.com).**

Another important factor with breathing is that you should always breathe through your nose. That is what the nose is designed to do, so logically, you should use it to breathe. Your tissues, organs, and brain get more benefit this way.

Nitric oxide is found in your nose. When you breathe through the nose, a small quantity of this gas goes into your lungs. Nitric oxide is important in keeping balance in the body (homeostasis), as well as being a bronchodilator, a vasodilator, and an antibacterial agent that helps neutralize bacteria and germs.

So, try to always be conscious of breathing through the nose, even when exercising. With practice, you can nose breathe during high intensity interval training. Your nasal passages will expand after a while, and you will naturally breathe through the nose at all times.

The 4 – 7 – 8 Breath Exercise for a Health Benefit: Sit up straight. Place the tip of your tongue against the back of your front teeth, and keep it there through the whole process. Breathe in casually and normally through the nose to the count of 4. Hold your breath to the count of 7. Exhale through the nose to the count of 8 with the breath making some sound. That completes one complete breath. Repeat 3 more times for a total of 4 breaths. If you're inclined, you can do this more times during the day, but each time, no more than the four breaths. After a month, you can up this to 8 breaths, which will be sufficient.

Breath Exercises for a Quick Energy Boost: These are two simple breathing exercises that will give you an instant energy boost. You might want to do them morning, noon, and early evening. But don't do them more than three times a day.

1. At the end of each out breath, there is a slight pause during which time carbon dioxide builds up. If you extend this pause, this buildup increases and causes you to inhale deeper on your next breath,

thereby pulling more oxygen into your system.

Here's the exercise. Breathe out, and at the end of the breath, tighten your stomach and force all the air out, pause for a count of six or eight, and then breathe in deeply through the nose. Do five of these breaths.

2. Separate, or immediately following the preceding exercise. Breathe in deeply through the nose, and on the out breath, through the mouth. As you are breathing out through the mouth, make the sound of 'aaah' half way through this out breath, and the sound of 'raaa' for the last half. Do three of these breaths, pause for ten seconds, three more, pause, and three more, for a total of nine.

Concentration

Concentration is important in any endeavor, especially exercise. Mind concentration centers your nerve energies and brings all your natural resources into play to intensify your muscular endeavors. The essence of concentration is focus. Try to bring total focus to each individual exercise or movement in your workout regimen. This will assimilate, coordinate, and fine-tune your breathing, movement, form, and timing. You gain a better overall sense of the exercise movements, which in turn enables you to function at top efficiency. Make it second nature.

Some Pertinent Other Points

Metabolism defines the processes that operate at the cellular level to change the body's stored fuel (predominately fat) into energy that operates the body, its chemistry, and keeps it warm. When someone says that their metabolism has slowed down now because they are older, they're not exactly right. Actually, most of your body energy comes from chemical processes that operate in your muscle tissue. Most people, as they age, lose muscle tissue unless they do something to fix the situation, such as exercise. A big key to losing fat and staying healthy is to create a larger metabolism by having an ample amount of lean muscle mass, because muscle is a great fat burner.

In general, long life depends on a lower metabolism. The less your systems have to work, the longer they will last, and the longer you can live. However, as we have mentioned, there are times, situations and reasons we need certain metabolic activity to increase. When metabolism is increased by exercise, it excites and activates hormonal activity in the body. If done properly, and in the right amount, this can be beneficial. But, people that are exercising many times more than is necessary during the week are consistently promoting an increased metabolism and the attendant hormonal action, especially adrenaline. Prolonged, elevated adrenaline will produce several serious age-related problems. It increases arterial plaque deposits, increases bad LDL cholesterol, ups the blood's tendency to clot, and lessens the body's ability to get rid of cholesterol. It also slows digestive secretions, and muscular movement of the gastrointestinal tract.

Men: Forget about all those hyped products that supposedly raise your testosterone levels. Just by bringing your waistline down from the 40+inch range to the low 30-inch range could increase testosterone levels by 50%. That 10 pounds of belly can reduce testosterone levels by half.

Body fat gain can cause testosterone to be converted to female hormone estrogen. A higher level of estrogen can turn off certain mechanisms that signal the body to make more testosterone. Estrogen and testosterone compete for body receptor sites, so you want to reduce estrogen. Some foods that can actually reduce testosterone are the sweetener Stevia, licorice, and grapefruit, along with alcohol, an estrogen producer.

Two supplements, Astaxanthin and Saw Palmetto, show an ability to get rid of some excess estrogen. Foods that are natural testosterone boosters: Beef, broccoli, chicken, oysters, cabbage, cauliflower, olive oil, mushrooms, wheat bran, and low fat yogurt. Cruciferous vegetables have a phytochemical called indole-3-cabinol (I3C) that helps rid the body of excess estrogen. Foods that have saturated fat and that have zinc are useful for testosterone production.

The digestion process of a pre-exercise meal close to a session can cause increased cortisol. And this can stifle your ability to burn fat and build muscle.

Some circles suggest that carbohydrates are not essential nutrients. However, they are important in certain functions. They are a source of fuel, and have important biological functions. A Severe and extended restriction of carbohydrates could lead to metabolic decline causing negative consequences on the body such as regeneration of tissue, growth and immunity, and other important processes. They activate an important process (PPP) that is necessary for the synthesis of DNA and RNA, along with ATP and NADPH (2 energy molecules). Factors associated with aging such as muscle deterioration and steroid hormone production are caused by the decrease of PPP that occurs with age. Carbs are relevant to growth hormone.

Digestive enzymes improve and offer support for muscle repair and growth due to their help with protein synthesis.

A man and a woman may weigh a certain weight when they are 25 years old. At 50 or 60 and older, they may say with pride that they still weigh the same as at 25, and assume they are fit and healthy. However, they are negating the fact that they have put on 6 to 10 inches around the waist and are softer. And a lot of shifting has taken place. Every inch is approximately 5 lbs, so, they have put on 30 or more pounds of fat and lost 30 or more pounds of muscle. They weigh the same, but they are not healthy and fit.

Abdominal fat (beer belly) is called visceral fat. It is dangerous in that it consistently releases inflammatory molecules into the body that significantly increases cancer risk, high blood pressure, heart disease, stroke, and other degenerative diseases. It also cramps and squeezes several important organs. Belly fat is a killer, and will shorten your life! Your waistline determines your quality of life. Sit-ups and all the rest without proper diet just build and tone the muscle over the abdominal fat. And, the most vigorous exercise will only burn 300 calories an hour. You can override this in just five minutes of eating junk. Proper nutrition and exercise are the only answers.

Your muscle tissue has elastic tissue surrounding them. Jumping into a program too fast or too heavy can cause microscopic tears and inflammation in this tissue. If you experience excessive muscle soreness or pain a day or two after exercising, make sure you drop back enough to eliminate this problem.

If you are over training, you will not feel good. Your brain will not get the glucose it requires, and it will not properly restore the glycogen in the muscles.

The power of the generative nerve supply is greatly dependent upon the condition of the neck. A strong neck gives you a great concentrated energy. Your neck is stronger than your arms. Push against your head with your hand and arm, and you will become aware of this. If you're capable, insert a neck bridge into your regimen.

The body cools itself by sweating. It does this more efficiently as your conditioning improves. Small dilating blood vessels send blood to the skin surface and radiate heat away from the body. There is an increase of a fluid and sodium mix from the sweat glands. As this evaporates, it causes a cooling of the body. Exercisers sweat more than others, but actually lose less salt. The body's cells re-absorb it as it moves from the sweat glands to the surface of the skin. Exercisers produce a greater volume of diluted sweat, which results in faster cooling.

You don't have to consume an excessive amount of protein to build muscles. But, to guard against performance loss as a result of decreased hormonal function you will want to eat well-balanced meals at the proper times, along with any necessary snacks, and adequate protein. Protein is the precursor for all hormones. Note: Craving sweets is a common sign of protein deficiency.

Don't consume carb drinks or sugary concoctions before a workout. This will alert the hypothalamus to relay a signal to the pancreas to up insulin and drop blood sugar levels. It will also alert the pituitary to signal the relative hormonal glands to hold back growth hormone. As you might surmise, if this happens, you have worked out for nothing.

If you stop exercising, your muscles will not turn to fat. They simply shrink because you have stopped your weight resistance training. Muscle and fat are two different things, and cannot turn into each other. Overeating, relative to your energy expenditure is the culprit.

Laughter should be considered as a healthy exercise. When we laugh, the brain and the body produce endorphins and enkephalins. Endorphins assist the immune system, and the production of T-cells is improved. The percentage of active ones are increased and made more energetic by enkephalins. Our internal organs are massaged by action produced by laughter.

Even if you have gone for many years without achieving a solid fitness and health level, remember, it is never too late. Sometimes reaching a goal after earlier misses can be an even greater achievement, and very rewarding.

Upon arising in the morning, you might want do a short 5 minute session of a few exercises found in **Yoga Compact (amazon.com).** Do them just after you get up. Also, If you do any type of morning workout, you can use them as a warm-up. It can also be used as a warm-up and a cool-down for any exercise session.

Here is something you might want to do for five minutes in the evening. This is an inverted yoga position that sends the blood from the extremities to your vital organs. It is especially good for the heart, lungs, and brain. It also reduces blood pressure.
Put some cushions next to a wall for a height of approximately one foot. Lie down with your butt on the cushions, and your legs up against the wall, perpendicular to your body. Relax, and breathe naturally. After you have worked with this position for a while, and if you are capable, you might want to try an inverted shoulder stand, or headstand.

There are certain exercises and breath techniques that can accentuate health in your subtle aspects. But only someone who has specific knowledge and understanding of these mechanisms should teach these. I offer these only by direct supervision in my **Yoga by Ennis** or **Ennis Life Science Regimen** sessions. Check the websites **(www.hleproductions.com or www.selfhelplifestyle.com)** periodically for listings of any new information or publications.

Modes and Programs

I have experimented with most of the exercise protocols found in the western part of the planet, and a few exotic ones from the far corners. Each of them has its claim to fame, and the famous advertise some of them. We have infomercials touting a great many of them. We have bodybuilding and weightlifting gurus, along with an array of resistance apparatus to purchase. We have various aerobics classes. There are several celebrity videos to go along with the numerous outdated Richard Simmons tapes. We have step aerobics, jazzercise, and aerobic routines utilizing Latin dance movements. We have tae bo. This uses martial arts movements, or broken kata, as its format. We have Pilates. We have yoga Pilates. We have the Power Gym people recommending this particular piece of equipment as a tool to do Pilates with. We have various forms of Yoga. And they all have certain benefits. But to use any one of them alone is too limiting.

Some of these promote strength way above aerobic conditioning; some promote aerobic conditioning at the expense of strength, and some create a blend of both. And some are harmful.

Resistance exercise done alone, not only produces physical strength, but also an aerobic effect if done properly. But generally, it doesn't produce as much aerobic benefit as we should have. In turn, Aerobic exercise will not produce brute strength in a sufficient amount. These two types of exercise may have a range of motion benefit if proper form is used, but a stretching series should be done along with them.

General yoga is especially touted for its alignment of the spine and flexibility. But for the results I desire, and the time constraints I need to impose, it falls a little short in the strength and aerobic category. Power Yoga, on the other hand, will produce both a strength and aerobic benefit higher than general yoga, and a stretch benefit, but still not enough overall.

We want to induce health, muscularity, strength, stamina, and flexibility as a by-product of our exercise choices. A balanced mixture of conditioning gives a better overall result for the average person. And it doesn't create sameness in your routine.

My choices are bodyweight exercises, cable exercises, weights and certain power yoga sequences; and aerobic conditioning such as high intensity interval training using running, jumping rope, bike intervals, and swimming in the ocean in the summertime, along with some run and sprint segments, and sometimes I enjoy a good walk. Put a combination of these together and you've got dynamite. For me, this combo gives me better overall results than anything I've ever done.

There are a multitude of variations you can use in bodyweight resistance, cables, and aerobics sessions. This lends to creativity and takes away from boredom. And the constant use of the power yoga sun salutation sequences is oil that will keep the conditioning effects of the other two coordinated. This combination also lends to excellent flexibility.

If you are a person who has a labor-intensive job, you might want to tailor your routine to suit your needs. A five-day format gives the less active person a daily injection of activity.

Changing your routine around at times will produce a somewhat different result. However, do not jump from one to the other during any given weekly routine. It may result in over-training, fatigue, or even injury. Finish up your current routine and start something different on a Monday.

I also recommend the relaxation exercise at the end of each daily session.

Some of you will be inclined to do more than the average person when it comes to exercise, due to the fact that it is something you really like to do.

Do your routine with enough intensity to keep you in an all-round good condition If you find your routine is a bit much for you, for one reason or another, feel free to scale it down. Experiment, and choose what empowers you and makes you feel good. Take your time. If you can't do all of one particular exercise, do what you can. Eventually, you will build up to a satisfying load and pace. You are not competing with anyone when you exercise, although at some point you may want to compete with yourself to see if you can better your effort.

Intense anaerobic routines are not recommended in starting out, because, unless each individual is brought to a competent level before starting to use these techniques, there may be problems.

An in-depth routine should require direct supervision as to manner and form. For my trainer sessions, I assess your individual needs, and construct ongoing routine changes relating to you directly about your diet, general health and lifestyle. Along with the tailored program, I also present a side workout of self-defense techniques, and at certain intervals, I present some special exercises that affect the subtle energy systems. These are only introduced in designed programs I personally supervise, and are only presented after some experience in meditation and mastering some specific breathing exercises.

My basic personal program always includes a routine of resistance exercise, high intensity interval training, and interspersed at times with some power yoga, jumping rope, abdominal work, along with biking, walking, run/sprint, etc. However, I will readily jump at the chance to play some volleyball, basketball, baseball, Frisbee, pin the tail on the donkey, or any other activity.

Be sure to use variety in your training program. This is called periodization. You risk possible damage to your musculoskeletal system by continually doing the same routine over and over. A periodic change-up keeps everything more invigorating.

It is generally advocated that you work out every other day, and rest the day in-between. I have found that once I am use to a daily program, which is varied in it's format, and leaves the week-end for rest, if you so choose, keeps me more invigorated. Also, as you get older, it is advocated that you exercise some every day to lessen the susceptibility of many debilitating diseases.

The time of day you workout is also important because your level of cortisol rises and falls as the day progresses. Cortisol is a natural hormone that raises metabolism along with body temperature, and readies the body to work. Cortisol also stimulates us to wake up from sleep when it is activated / released by light exposure, low blood sugar levels and other factors. Exercise lends to activation. Cortisol levels start to activate at sunrise, peak between 9:00 a.m. and 12:00 p.m., and decrease during the afternoon. By 6:00 p.m. daily output is done, and this makes it easier to wind down and eventually go to sleep.

Some major sports authorities say that when cortisol levels are highest, one can naturally train better. They also believe that training after work in the early evening may cause sleep disruption and disrupt the recovering / repair cycles. The physical repair cycle is between 10 p.m. and 2 a.m. The psychological repair cycle is between 2 a.m. and 6 a. m. This disrupting can cause you to wake up feeling lethargic.

As noted, exercise lends to the activation of cortisol. So, if you work out in the evening, the body gets the feeling it is in the timeframe between sunrise and midday. Essentially, you will be winding yourself up for the night. When cortisol is released, it lasts for hours before it dissipates. If released in the evening, it will still be active at bedtime. This can keep you from getting a deep, or restorative sleep.

Note. If you work out in the evening, but still sleep good, this may suggest an underlying problem of fatigued adrenal glands. You're sleeping good because the released cortisol from exercise is bringing the adrenals back up to a baseline functioning. A problem is being covered.

The ability to do your exercise routine between 9 and 12 in the morning is impractical for most people. But, if you can do it then, you will be in the ideal time frame. Otherwise, try to workout as early as you can in the late afternoon, as opposed to the early evening.

A resistance routine should take 20 minutes to 40 minutes (give or take), including the warm-up and cool down, and depending on the routine for a particular day. An aerobic session should be a high intensity interval session of 20 minutes, and generally performed on an alternate day of resistance exercise.

Stretch only after any workout because the body is warm and therefore more easily stretched. It is also complimentary to the lifting routine. Do stretches that affect your legs and back. The book **Yoga Compact (Amazon.com)** illustrates the sun salutations and other flexibility exercises. Whatever type of stretching you do, make sure to start out slow and easy. Do not hold any stretch in a pain zone, as this can produce microscopic tears.

Your weekly routine should produce power, strength, endurance, flexibility, and balance. Experiment with interchanging some of the exercises. Create variations in the routine as to sequence and etc. Design, and mix-n-match the exercises and scheduling in a way that suits you personally. Whatever you favor, the most important thing is to get at it!

After exercising, particularly in the late afternoon, if you meditate, you might want to do so as soon as possible because, at this time you should be calm, relaxed, and centered.

Don't get dehydrated during your exercise period. Drink a glass of water one half hour before you work out, and drink a glass five minutes after you're finished. Note: If you sweat profusely, and you consume an excessive amount of water immediately after you finish, it may cause excessive urination, and in the process be dehydrating.

Example of a Basic Weekly Routine

This is just to give you an example of a weekly routine. We will use a warm-up, a cool-down, pull-ups, bodyweight squats, push-ups, and running wind sprints as the example exercises. However, if you do this routine, and continue to increase your reps and degree of resistance by variation each week, you will get a very good result. You can start any day you choose. I will use Monday as the start example. I assume that most people are familiar with these basic resistance exercises. However, if you have just arrived from planet 'Don't Know', here are descriptions.

Basic Pull-up: Done by hanging from a bar higher than your overhead reach. Use a shoulder width grip, with the hand palms facing away from you. Take a breath, and on the out breath, pull you body up until your chin is even with the bar, and then, breathing in, lower yourself back to the start position and repeat.

Basic Bodyweight squat: Stand straight with your hands up at shoulder height, palms forward, as if someone was holding a gun on you. Position the feet shoulder width apart, with the toes angled out slightly. Breathing in, squat down fully with your back straight, but naturally, slightly forward, as in sitting down in a chair. Pause, ever so slightly. Breathing out, push yourself back up, with a prominent amount of thrust through the heels of your feet, until you are up straight, and repeat.

Basic Push-up: Get down on all fours. Position yourself with your hands on the floor, shoulder width apart, and with the arms extended. Your head should be straight, in line with the body, as a straight stick. The feet are close together, or barely apart. Breathing in, lower your body until the upper arms are at right angles with the lower arms, or further down with the nose at the floor. Breathing out, push yourself back up to the starting position. Repeat.

Monday – Wednesday - Friday: Resistance exercise: Your choice of a 5-10 minute warm-up, followed by two sets of however many pull-up repetitions you can perform. Do anywhere from 1 to 5 pull-ups for set one, depending on ability. Rest 30 seconds to a minute between set 1 and set 2, depending on your conditioning. Do second set of pull-ups. After set 2, rest for one minute and then start the bodyweight squats. Do one set of ten or fifteen, rest 30 seconds to a minute, and do another set of 10 or 15. Rest for one minute or more as needed, and move to the push-ups. Do one set of 1,3,5,10, or 15, depending on ability, rest 30 seconds to a minute, then do another set of push-ups. At the end of the push-up segment, do a 5-minute cool-down. You can end your exercise session at this point, or you may want to do the relaxation exercise described previously.

Tuesday – Thursday: High intensity interval session: Do five minutes of walking for a warm-up, followed by a session that last for no longer than 20 minutes total time, including rest time, and finish with a five minute walk as a cool-down. Here are two ways to do this. Here is the first way: Walk for five minutes. Then do a slow pace run or jog to be interspersed with 6 or 7 wind sprints. The wind sprints should be fast, but not all-out. After each wind sprint segment, drop back to the slow run, or jog, until your breathing returns to normal, then sprint again. Do this procedure until you have filled in 20 minutes of time. Then, walk for 5 minutes to finish off the session. Here is the second way: Warm up with five minutes of walking. Now, sprint all-out, as fast as you can, until you have to stop and catch your breath. At this time, and no matter how long it takes, walk, or stop completely, until your breathing returns to normal. Repeat the all out sprint, walk/stop to normal breathing sequence, until you have used up 20 minutes. Walk for 5 minutes as your cool-down. The end. Start with an intensity level that is comfortable, and progress.

You can use the above weekly routine examples to great effect by upping the reps and using harder variations for the resistance segments, and by increasing the intensity of the interval sessions. You can use this methodology by using bodyweight exercises, lifting weights, using cable band exercises, or any type resistance exercise. You just increase the resistance and score the reps as your progress will allow. High intensity interval sessions are adaptable to running, riding a bike, using a treadmill, swimming, rowing, jumping rope, or any relative exercise.

The Weeks-end

You might want to participate in weekend sports or other activities such as biking, hiking, walking, swimming in the lake or ocean, etc. I suggest doing the yoga Sun Salutations right on through the weekend. Or you may rest. Your energy level should determine your actual output. According to your energy and desire, you may want to go dancing. Dancing is the only art form that the artist can become one with. Therefore, it is a form of meditation. The painter can't become the picture, or the musician the music, but the dancer becomes the dance. I dance every weekend, sometimes during the week. Dancing is one of the great elixirs of life. It's great exercise, great fun, and a great stress buster. It's almost impossible to be unhappy when you're on the dance floor. My dance of choice is the Carolina shag. Oh, the metaphysics of shag.

Note: At this writing, I reside in the Ocean Drive (OD) section of North Myrtle Beach, S.C. This is the Mecca for shag aficionados. If you're ever in the neighborhood, check out Ducks, Fat Harold's Beach Club, the Pavilion, the Pirate's Cove, the Spanish Galleon, and the OD Arcade, along with the week-long SOS dance and party events held twice a year.

What to Eat Relative to Exercise

Let's start out by presenting what not to eat before, during, or after an exercise session. Avoid sports drinks, energy drinks, energy bars, protein bars, and the like, because they contain sugar, and usually fructose. These will undo the exercise benefits. Fructose has been shown to lend to abdominal obesity (belly fat), to decrease HDL, increase LDL, elevate triglycerides, raise blood sugar, raise blood pressure, and more. Having a recovery drink or meal with high sugar within two hours of working out will negate the effects of exercise relative to human growth hormone production.

You may be unaware that it is best to workout on an empty stomach. Although, at least try to wait 2-3 hours after a meal. However, if exercising on an empty stomach makes you feel weak or sick feeling, you can eat a small meal a half an hour before the session, preferably a fast acting protein such as whey protein (15-20g) to curb your appetite. Whey protein before and after a resistance workout session can build muscle and burn fat simultaneously.

Exercise performed on an empty stomach helps prevent weight gain and insulin resistance. The sympathetic nervous system (SNS) controls the fat burning processes of the body, and exercise, along with no food activates the SNS. This combo promotes the breakdown of fat and glycogen for energy, and necessitates fat burning.

When exercise and fasting, such as intermittent fasting are combined, certain genes and growth factors are activated that recycle and rejuvenate muscle and brain tissue. It alerts the body to keep the brain, the neuro-motors and muscle fibers biologically young. Note: Use intermittent fasting only 1 or 2 times per week.

Note: Intermittent fasting generally means that you eat your evening meal, and you don't eat again until the next day's evening meal. This type fasting can normalize your insulin sensitivity, normalize the hunger hormone (ghrelin) levels, promote human growth hormone (HGH) production, lower triglyceride levels, reduce free radical damage, and reduce inflammation. Some studies indicate that it may enhance immune function, decrease blood pressure, increase lifespan, protect against cardiovascular disease, neurodegenerative disorders, and cancer.

Your post workout meal *after a resistance session* is very important. It sends nutrients to repair and grow muscle tissue. In order to feed the muscle before tearing down begins, you need to eat some fast-assimilating protein such as whey protein and a fast released carbohydrate, such as a banana to replace glycogen within 30 minutes after a workout. You can eat your main meal at a later time. You need to replace the glycogen storage in your muscles fairly soon after an exercise session, or caloric consumption may be deposited as fat. Glycogen replenishment is said to be doubled if you eat sooner rather than waiting a couple of hours. This is also said to produce a more raised level of testosterone and growth hormone. Note: If you eat white flour products, or sugar, you may feel listless during your workout. The body uses more energy to push these food sources through your system. Sugar also tends to leave your muscles stiff.

The time to eat *after an aerobic/cardio session* such as a high intensity interval training session should be 30-45 minutes. That gives the body time to utilize the fat burning effect. Waiting more than an hour to eat will begin to slow your metabolism.

Ideally, you should then eat a protein source of meat, poultry, or fish, along with a vegetable-type of carbohydrate.

Sleep

Balance in our outer activities is represented by the figure 8. Eight hours of service or work, eight hours of recreation (re-creation), and eight hours of rest and sleep. To make your exercise program beneficial, make sure you get plenty of quality rest and sleep, so your body can repair and rebuild, and your mind can rest from the activities of the day.

If you catch only a few hours of sleep on a regular basis it can inhibit metabolism and hormone production in a manner akin to the effects of early stage diabetes and aging. The disruption of the sleep/wake cycle (circadian rhythm) may affect cancer progression.

The energy absorbed from food is not transferred directly while you are eating. It is transferred during sleep. If you eat a large meal close to bedtime, energy has to be diverted from the physical regeneration period of sleep (slow wave sleep-10 p.m. to 2 a.m.) where secretions of growth hormone occur to work on digestion. The later hours of sleep (REM) can be seen as a psychic repair time.

If you have a sleep debt, or you get a drop in your alertness after lunchtime, you might want to catch an hour of sleep after lunch. This will boost your energy and alertness for the rest of the day, and take an hour off your sleep debt. Of course, you may not have an hour to burn after lunch. If not, fifteen minutes spent lying on your left side will aid digestion and give you a charge for your afternoon activities.

Sleep increases energy, boosts immunity, and boosts Natural Killer Cells. After only a few hours of sleep loss, you start to lose a considerable amount of immunity to disease. Note. Meat eaters and people who have jobs that require a lot of mental activity need more sleep. Also. Don't take the sleep drugs you see advertised. They interfere with REM (rapid eye movement) sleep. This is the time we relax most deeply, and dream. Loss of REM sleep can cause you to overeat during the day, and can contribute to high blood pressure. If you are meditating, eating properly, and getting sufficient exercise, you are not going to have any problem sleeping.

Check This Out! Spirit as Personal Trainer

Check this out! You can have the Holy Spirit (Divine Kundalini) as your personal trainer, but only if you meditate, and have reached the point where you have a direct experience of the Presence during meditation. You can ask it to give you a perfect exercise regimen for the day. To do this, sit down, get into your quiet meditative state, and call for the Holy Spirit to anoint you with its presence. When this happens, ask it to give you the proper workout for the day. Sit still, and wait for the activity to start. You will know when the divine routine is over by the cessation of the activity.

The routine may be of long or short duration, depending upon your needs. In my case, I can designate a time frame and the session will end then. I have noticed that if I had any discordant condition at the time, such as a leg or shoulder problem, the routine would address and straighten them out. After a while, you intuitively know when to mix and match your regular workout with the divine workout. There have been times when I would opt for the divine routine and nothing would happen. I would then do my regular workout for the day, and at the end of it I would sit for the Holy Spirit, and some divine movements would top off my regular workout. At other times I would opt for the divine, and at the end I would know to go forward with my regular routine for the day. For my part, I have come to feel that I am expected to do my routine, and that the Holy Spirit will add its exercises as need be. A good approach would be to ask the Holy Spirit to lead, guide, and direct you in your exercise program.

All exercise helps relieve stress, but the personal sessions with the Presence produce a dramatic stress release. Experiment with this concept. Note:

Make sure you sit still long enough for the Presence to start your routine. It must receive your serious intention for it to activate in this particular endeavor.

You will know if this protocol speaks to you. If you wish to expand your consciousness relative to this scenario, read the books **Infinity of Intrigue** or **Life is a Science, Not a Roll of the Dice (amazon.com).** I offer life science protocols through individual sessions, or by seminar.

Conclusion

As you can tell, I take my exercise seriously. Not to do so is tantamount to slow suicide. This is one of the prerequisites to living a full life. Determine to master your fitness plan by knowledge, control, consistency, and pride. Make this area of your life a discipline and lifetime habit. It will stand you in good stead for the rest of your earthy sojourn.

Inertia bogs us down in triviality, and stagnates a proper and joyous unfolding in all areas of our lives. So, be active with your physical body.

If your day consists of adequate physical exercise, good nutrition, and a time for meditation, you will automatically rise above the thundering herd. Make these three disciplines a mandatory part of your life each day. Approach them seriously in your intention to carry them out, and with positive expectation and joy in your application.

I hope that the information presented may have offered you some refreshment on your journey through life. A toast goes to all who are dedicated to the quest for better health and fitness.

_____ HLE _____
Harrison Langdon Ennis

Author Services and Products

If you found **Exercise Exposed** to be informative and enlightening and wish to have a compact, well-rounded, illustrated regimen at your disposal, you may want to get **Yoga Compact (amazon.com).** If you are interested in personal training, life science protocols, or consultation, use the email address below.

HLE continues to offer sites that reel in a lifetime of learning and creating. They provide knowledge, service, and products on a variety of interests that point to a passion for life. Take a closer look for a spark to widen your horizons as you pass through your present life stream. Check the following sites regularly for updates.

Websites:

HLE Productions: www.hleproductions.com

Self Help Lifestyle: www.selfhelplifestyle.com

Amazon.com for **Harrison Langdon Ennis**

Check above sites periodically for new additions.

Email: contact@hleproductions.com

"Be a legend in your own mind, and then try to live up to it." HLE